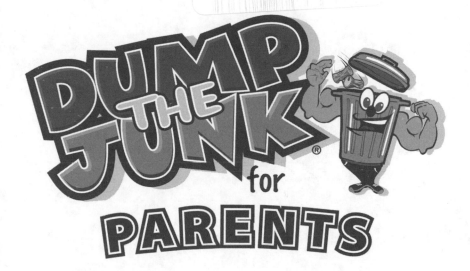

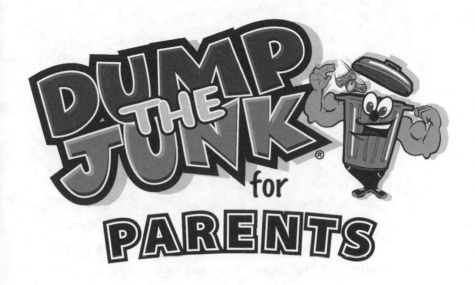

THE ANSWER TO CHILDHOOD OBESITY

DR. JOSEPH CHRISTIANO

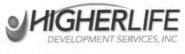

DEVELOPMENT SERVICES, INC

Oviedo, Florida

Dump the Junk for Parents—The Answer to Childhood Obesity
by Dr. Joseph Christiano

Published by HigherLife Development Services, Inc.
400 Fontana Circle
Building 1 – Suite 105
Oviedo, Florida 32765
(407) 563-4806
www.ahigherlife.com

ISBN 13: 978-1-935245-36-0
ISBN 10: 1-935245-36-8

Cover Design: r2c Design—Rachel Lopez

First Edition

10 11 12 13 — 9 8 7 6 5 4 3 2 1

Printed in the United States of America

Dedication

I want to thank Diane Bolger, my 'Champion,' who was very instrumental in positioning me to move to Stockton, California, where I implemented the first Dump the Junk Curriculum for At-Risk and Obese High School students at Amos Alfonso Stagg H.S. Diane and husband Ed made my five-month stay possible.

For the development and publishing of this book, I thank all the staff at HigherLife. I thank Patti Reynolds, Sergeant at Arms, who gracefully handled all my questions and concerns and made them systematically smooth out. I thank Hope Flinchbaugh for her ability to translate what I wanted this book to say and Marsha McCoy for staying on top of the production of this project.

Of course, for the success of this and every book I have written, a loving 'thank you' goes without saying to Lori, my wife for her endless support and driving force.

Last but not least, I thank my creator and God, Yahweh, who, as I specialize in the field of health and fitness, reminds me over and over of His incredible creative work, the human body.

Special Dedication

I thank my dear friend who shared the same passion as me for helping our kids be healthy, Belinda Higgins, who is not here to see the publishing of this book or the Dump the Junk K-4 Whole-Health Curriculum. My loving memories of "Mz. B" will always be cherished.

Table of Contents

Introduction

MY NAME IS DR. Joe Christiano, I'm a naturopathic doctor and health and fitness life coach. I have trained Hollywood actors as well as swimsuit winners in the Miss USA, Miss America, and Mrs. America Pageants.

I can tell you that no matter what your career, good nutrition, physical fitness, and a positive self-image begin during childhood, at home. It's true what they say—home is where the heart is. And home is where good health starts. This small handbook will give you tips on how to lead your family in three vital areas:

1. **Attitude—Think up!**
2. **Exercise—Power up!**
3. **Nutrition—Fill up!**

Grocery shopping.
Somebody has to do it. Food industries make all sorts of promises, but few deliver the food choices that are best for our kids. How do you choose? How do you dump the junk and collect the wholesome?

Nutrition is sometimes the most difficult aspect to navigate. It's difficult to plot a course through the thousands of choices in today's grocery store. The question is this—how can we really tell which food packages are living up to those "healthy" promises, especially for our kids?

Take this book with you next time you shop. Check out my kids' snacks list (in the back) and compare it to what you normally buy. Don't worry—I did my best to be kid-friendly. No carrot juice suggested. Walk with me through the grocery store, and I'll help you dump the junk and bring home the very best food for your family.

And remember, getting fit is not just about biceps and waistlines. Being fit has much to do with your mental attitude about yourself. You are very valuable, and your child is priceless, created for pleasure and joy. Come on. Let's get started.

Section 1

Attitude
Think Up!

Obstacles are those frightful things you see when you take your eyes off your goal.

—Henry Ford[1]

Section 1

Attitude

Think Up!

THINK ABOUT IT—WHAT WOULD stop in your life if you lost your health? Everything.

I'm here to help you plan for what's most valuable to you—your life and the life of your child. Good health habits begin at home. Think about it— what nutritional habits (good or bad) did you pick up from your parents when you were a child?

My sweet Italian mother just loved to feed her family! I remember coming home from school in the middle of winter, and on the kitchen table were twelve pans of the most scrumptious, delicious homemade bread, butter melting down the sides. I stood there with my tongue hanging out. Ma would ask proudly, "Joey, would you like a piece of bread?" Before I could answer, she would hack off a wedge about three inches thick, lather it with butter, and thrust it into my hands.

Every day we ate her gourmet Italian dishes made from scratch—pasta, ravioli, gnocchi, chicken cacciatore, and that wonderful homemade bread.

My father, a man of few words, had only one rule at the supper table: "Take all you want, but eat all you take." It didn't take long for the four of us kids to learn how to pack it away.

> **The U.S. Surgeon General has declared obesity to be a national health epidemic.**[2]

I used to eat twice as much as my brothers and sisters. All my relatives heard about how much I could eat. Why, a big eater like me made the front page of the *Italian Gazette*! I got a pat on the back for eating like a pig.

When I was a kid, I burned up all those calories playing, but as a young adult, I grew to a huge 305 pounds!

The good news is that I dropped more than 85 pounds, won the Mr. Florida title, and later took the first runner-up in the Mr. USA contest and fourth runner-up in Mr. America. What made the difference?

It started with attitude. I had to keep my eyes on the purpose, not the task.

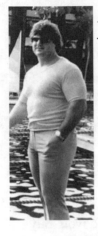

Before Photo—
305 lbs, April 1981

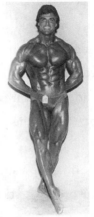

After Photo—
220 lbs, December 1981

Focus on the Purpose Not the Task

Today, as a health and fitness life coach, I've learned that children and teenagers will model the food, fitness, and attitude choices that they see at home. I'm not implying that we should mold (or scold) kids into our image, but we can provide them the cement in their foundation to discover who they are in this world. That begins with positive affirmation. Your child can flourish into the picture of good health with your encouragement.

Parents and children sometimes encounter speed bumps that slow us down in our goals to become fit. Speed bumps are normal; just don't allow yourself to be overwhelmed by the task in front of you. Look at the goal ahead. In order to reach your goal, you will need to stay focused on that goal. This is the type of attitude that will carry you when you aren't sure you can go any farther, or when everything and everyone has failed you.

Imagine a soccer field as your family's field of fitness. In order to stay healthy as a family, you have to set boundaries or limitations on the food you buy, the portion sizes you serve your child, and the amount of time you allow him or her to play video games or watch TV. Those boundaries are good. They keep everyone in the family on the field of fitness. If a family member goes out of bounds, don't sweat it. Just throw the ball back into the field, get back in the game of family fitness, and keep your eyes on the goal. That's the winning attitude!

Although we don't always think about it, we live within boundaries every day. What about school? Every child in the United States under the age of seventeen is required to go to school. No options. We can all remember times when we felt we couldn't go any farther, we were tired, and we didn't want to do our homework. Lucky for us, our government mandates the boundaries in the "field" of education. Because those boundaries are there, our child has to "get on the field" and go to school. Our children need the similar boundaries when it comes to staying healthy. And parents are the ones to provide those boundaries. If we model healthy choices and insist on exercise and nutrition, our children will come up to the high goals that we set for them.

Here's the secret: *Focus on the purpose, not the task.*

Make this statement your personal mantra. Hang it on the fridge. Tape it to your dashboard. Better yet, tuck it into your child's book bag. *Focus on the purpose, not the task.*

Does your pediatrician have one of those posters hanging in the office? "101 Ways to Praise A Child." I'm sure you know that a parent's words are powerful. A parent's words have the power to enable a child to overcome any speed bump on the pathway to health. Here are a few words of praise that will encourage your child to focus on the purpose, not the task:

- You're a winner!
- I believe in you!
- You're the best!
- Looking good!
- Excellent job!
- Way to go!
- Outstanding!
- You are a treasure!
- You're sensational!
- You're beautiful!
- I knew you could do it!

> **Focus on the purpose, not the task.**

These are words that will help your child leap over the tasks in front of them and make it to the goal line of physical fitness and health. Repeat these words of empowerment when you wake up in the morning, during the day, and before you go to bed at night. Remind your kids to do the same.

This repetitious mental exercise will allow your subconscious to receive these empowering words over and over, and over time you will develop the mental "stay power" to push through the tasks necessary for reaching any of your goals.

The Original "Can Man"

I'm known today as "Dr. Joe, the Can Man." That's because I tell kids everywhere to dump the junk (into the can) so they can live a healthy life. But this "Can Man" nickname actually has a double meaning. And my story has everything to do with focusing on the purpose—not the task.

At the age of twenty-five, I had tried several different employment opportunities, but wasn't satisfied. I had a desire to help people be healthier, so I decided to become a health professional—a goal that was not that simple.

Dump the Negative Thoughts!

1. I Can't
2. I'm a Loser
3. I Don't Care

There were several obstacles or tasks to deal with. I knew I wanted to move to Florida, establish a new career, and feed my family of five. Since my employment at the time paid me two hundred dollars per week, I had plenty of motivation to do what was needed. But what could I do to overcome this tremendous challenge to move and make my dream come true?

I was employed at a major sanitation company in western New York. I was a sales rep and sold heavy-duty compactors and waste management equipment—those big cardboard compactors you see in the back of the stores in the malls and shopping centers. Soon I was operations manager there.

I noticed most of the guys who worked at the waste management center were anywhere from eighteen years old to my age of twenty-five. But there happened to be one guy who was fifty-five years old and looked extremely weather beaten, tired, and weary. His name was Don.

I felt bad for Don. I asked him how he was doing one day and he replied that he was dead tired. I asked him why he was still on the back of the G-truck throwing garbage everyday when all the other workers were so much younger than he was. He told me that when he and the owner of the company were kids, the owner wanted to start a sanitation company and told Don if Don would start with him, he would take good care of Don. Well, his old friend and owner of this huge sanitation company forgot Don over the years, and consequently Don was stuck on the back of a truck with failing hopes of his friend's promise. My next question was, "If you could do it all over again, what would you do?"

He looked at me and said, "If I were thirty years younger (that was my age, by the way), I would start my own garbage company, grow it, and then sell it and move to where the weather is warm."

A light as clear as daylight came on—I was that twenty-five-year-old younger guy! At that very moment I made a decision to become one—A Can Man!

I knew the business. I had learned the ropes but never was on the back of a truck nor ever wanted to be. This huge task that I was about to take on was not at all my idea of making a career change but instead was a means to get me there. In my mind all I saw were those sandy beaches, beautiful swaying palm trees, no more snowy, ice-cold winters, and becoming a natural health professional: my goal!

My parents supported my decision and helped me by co-signing a small loan so I could buy my first truck.

When I urge you to *focus on the purpose, not the task*, I know from first-hand experience what I am saying because there were plenty of "tasks" for which I hadn't planned.

I recall those frozen winter days when I had to wake up at 4 A.M. and shovel my way out of the driveway just to get out on the road, and then drive to the yard where my truck was. Once there, I had to try to start a frozen truck engine, and if I could without needing a jumpstart, I could begin my day. After fighting blizzard conditions, climbing snow banks to get to my customers' garbage cans, freezing my fingers off, and not having any flat tires or accidents, I would return home by midnight. Or how about those hot summer days when the garbage smelled so terrible I could vomit? Or the time I dumped a can in the back of the truck and the soupy garbage with maggots splashed back into my face? *Tasks, tasks, tasks!*

> ## Overcome the task and focus on the future.

As my company grew, so did the hours, workload, and tasks for this Can Man. Do you think I wasn't challenged with keeping that "stay power" attitude? Let's face it, I was doing something for four long years I really didn't want to be doing. When the tasks became overwhelming, I made myself look at the future and where I was going, not where I was.

Finally, I reached my goal! I sold my business and moved to Florida. Today, I own a natural health and fitness company, I am a naturopathic doctor, and I am absolutely enjoying the fruits from a mantra I learned to use many years ago: *focus on the purpose, not the task.*

So when the going gets somewhat challenging and the kids are not getting with the program, don't let their negative opposition or lack of participation on their part destroy your opportunity of reaching your goals as a healthy family. You can do it!

Stay Focused

Have you ever watched the Kentucky Derby or other famous horse races on television? If so, you have probably noticed the blinders on the outside of each horse's eyes. The purpose of these blinders is to prevent the horse from being distracted by anything that comes into view on either side of his head. The horse's owner and trainers realize how important it is to keep the animal focused. The same is true here.

Maintaining focus helps us to lead our family in a positive way, perhaps like never before. Don't let any distractions keep you from achieving what you want to accomplish for your kids. Let them dream their dreams, set their goals, and show them how much you believe in them as you lead the way.

I Don't Care Attitude Says:

- I don't think very much of myself.
- I don't deserve anything good in life.
- I'm just not smart enough.
- I do not deserve to be healthy.
- I let others treat me with disrespect because I don't respect myself.
- I accept being a loser in life.

I Care Attitude Says:

- I believe in myself.
- I care about myself.
- I respect myself.
- I deserve the best in life.
- I am worth taking care of.
- I am a winner by choice.

Self-control and Setting Boundaries— Combat Twins for Protection

I count him braver who overcomes his desires than him who conquers his enemies; for the hardest victory is over self.

—Aristotle (Greek Philosopher)[3]

Setting boundaries and applying self-control are two very powerful strengths you can use to protect yourself and your children from a myriad of negative assailants, both from within and without. Believe it or not, you do *not* have to allow these assailants to reside within you:

- Overindulgence
- Uncontrolled desires
- Impulsive decision-making habits
- Backsliding into former habits that cause failure
- An abusive relationship
- Never learning to set boundaries as a child and today struggling with eating disorders
- Low self-esteem

There is hope.

As an adult, much of what your caretakers taught you as a child affects your thinking process today. This is why you as the parent must come to grips with these concepts so you can instill them into your young sons and daughters.

Self-control—Protecting Me from Myself!

Your power to apply self-control will serve as your personal bodyguard, protecting you from *yourself*. It won't matter what or who your assailant is—overcoming emotional eating, overeating, overspending what your budget allows—changing your attitude about your self-worth and having self-control puts you in the driver seat so you can reach your destiny.

As this starts making sense to you on a personal level, you will see how your children will benefit from your example as they face their Goliath at school, with friends, and making adult decisions.

If a person did not learn how to set boundaries in the formative years, this person can eventually grow into adulthood with eating disorders such as compulsive eating, anorexia, bulimia, and overeating, all of which are often connected to a lack of boundaries.

> **Self-control builds confidence.**

Let me share a scenario with you about a grown woman with an eating disorder. When Susie was an eight- or nine-year-old girl, she kept a diary of the events of her day in her personal journal. One day when Susie was not home, her brother and a couple of his friends happened to go into her bedroom and found her diary. The boys opened the diary and started reading all of the events, feelings, and personal thoughts that Susie had recorded. The boys were laughing and having fun with the diary when Susie walked into the room. Needless to say, the boys knew they were wrong. But instead of confronting her brother and his friends, Susie just sat on her bed and cried. She never did anything about it. Instead, she let those hurt feelings stay deep inside.

> **If you don't believe you
> have self-worth or value,
> what is there to protect?**

Had Susie been taught how to set boundaries, she would have gotten in her brother's face, told him a thing or two, and snatched her book out of his hand. Had she done that, her actions would have been based on personal standards she was taught to set as to what she thought about herself. In essence, her reaction to her brother would have reinforced her sense of self-value and self-worth. She would have known that her brother was not allowed to violate those standards without consequence. Had boundaries been in place, her brother would have been more apprehensive about reading her diary in the future. But most importantly, Susie would have had developed a healthy sense of self-love and self-value instead of an eating disorder as a grown woman.

Think about this for a minute: *If you don't believe you have self-worth or value, what is there to protect?*

Teach your kids how valuable they are and how to protect themselves from those who would abuse or take advantage of them.

Boundaries and Forgiveness

"I love you, but...!"

Several years ago, I counseled a woman in her mid- to late forties. She was very attractive but her outward beauty was somewhat hidden because of her grossly overweight condition. She said she had tried everything. She had read up on all the latest exercise programs and diet plans, and she even took dietary supplements. "How could I make all these lifestyle changes, lose weight, and yet not be able to keep it off?" she asked.

After spending an hour or so with her I was able to determine her real struggle. I had noticed in her questionnaire that she mentioned as a pre-teen the fact that her mother was always on her case about her weight. She told me that if her mother walked through the door right now, she would ask, "When are you planning to lose all that weight?"

I posed a direct question to my client. I asked her whether she had forgiven her mother yet. And if she hadn't, she needed to.

The very moment I asked that question, I saw these huge tears of pent-up pain start flowing down her cheeks. I knew that I had hit the root of the problem. I told her she also needed to stop blaming her mother. As she was crying, I began to explain to her that all the knowledge in the world wouldn't help her lose weight and keep it off until she addressed the root problem. In her case it was an emotionally rooted problem—unforgiveness!

My recommendation was first to forgive her mother before she started to make any healthy lifestyle changes, or she would just be spinning her wheels. Her comment was, "My mother would never understand why I would want to forgive her because she would deny that she was the problem I was struggling with."

Her mother was never going to change. But I wanted my client to be free. I explained that it was her responsibility to heal and move on with her life. I told her by forgiving her mother, she would begin the healing process from the emotional pain she was suppressing all these years—she would be free!

Had my client been taught how to set boundaries as a young preteen girl, her mother's words would not have caused her all that pain. Her overweight condition was not her problem but rather a symptom of a root problem. Now in her forties, she had to learn that she had value and worth and learn the significance of setting boundaries.

> **Your goal is progress,
> not perfection.**

Self-control and learning to set boundaries are tasks you will need to develop and perfect. Your overall goal, however, is not to be perfect—but to make progress.

Teach your kids to set boundaries that will protect them from abusive people, harmful and abusive words, and expectations or peer pressure that they will face in life. This will translate to them if you teach them they have value and worth. You know that anything of value is worth protecting. Teach them the importance of self-control and they will think before they decide to do drugs, drink alcohol, or have sex.

Give them the opportunity to grow into what they are, and they will be all they can be. Make their home environment healthy and full of love.

Here are some tips on how to be their attitude coach at home.

Family-Friendly Attitudes

- Do you find yourself or any of your children making choices that are impulsive and without much thought? Consider whether your decision(s) are based on what you "ought to do" rather than a quick, flippant response. STOP and THINK before you respond or react to a situation, problem, or question.

> **Self-control is the power within to protect yourself from yourself.**

- People will invade your privacy, cross over the line, and violate you if you do not set boundaries for yourself. Set a high standard to live by. When we realize our value and worth, we will set boundaries that hold any abuser from within or without at the boundary line.

- Forgive others, including caretakers, for causing you emotional or physical pain. Not forgiving others contributes to a negative emotional condition and damaging physical health, over time. And eventually the pain turns into anger, and anger turns into bitterness. Forgiving is a means to set you free and the healing process can take place. If you find you cannot forgive someone—for whatever reason—you may want to think about seeking counseling.

> **Staying focused on the goal is the key to success.**

- Does your child find it difficult to finish or complete a given task? Yes or no? Cheer them on. Encourage them to stay focused. Be patient with them.

- In the process our vision can get a bit blurred, and consequently we lose focus of the intended target. If that is the case with your child, remind her to repeat our mantra—*focus on the purpose, not the task.* Remind him of the reasons *why* they chose that goal or the importance of completing it.

- Are you willing to do what it takes to accomplish your long-term goals and the goals for your kids? Yes or no? If yes, then view each task as a mere stepping stone for accomplishing the goals. Verbally support them as they need to be stretched.

- Many of us can get very excited and even motivated to make changes, especially after being pumped up by someone's success story. But once we jump into the water and find out how cold it is, we swim to the side to get out as fast as we can. Staying focused is the key to success.

Be positive with your kids. Make your kids as accountable to you as you are to them. Make the family-friendly attitude exercises a team thing. This will give them the sense of camaraderie that she or he is not in it alone. Write the mantra and tack it up on your fridge—focus on the purpose and not the task. Tell them that you believe in them. Encourage them to stay focused on the purpose, not the task.

As you implement these healthy lifestyle practices, keep them simple and remember to enjoy the journey. My hope and prayer for you is that you will provide your children with all the tools available to you so they can become champions in life.

Section 2

Nutrition
Fill Up!

Section 2

Nutrition

Fill Up!

WEIGHT CONTROL CAN BE a frustrating problem. Perhaps you're aware that the U.S. Surgeon General has declared obesity to be a national health epidemic. 31.9% of children and adolescents are overweight and 16.3% of children are obese in the United States.[4] Losing and keeping off the pounds can lead to desperation—in children, teens, and adults.

It's important not to slip into fad dieting in an effort to lose weight or to help your child lose weight. To accomplish a healthy weight we need to ignore quick weight-loss dieting gimmicks and apply some very simple practices that will last a lifetime.

Food Guilt

Do you feel pressured to diet? I'm sure you know the routine:

1. I'm good if I stick with the rules.
2. I'm bad if I blow it.

The people that I train and coach in health and fitness will sometimes show up on Monday morning and tell me, "I was bad this weekend."

I answer, "Really? Did you cheat on your husband?" No. They had a chocolate candy bar.

"Really? Well, guess what—you're not a sinner."

The dieting-it-off concept has ruined people. If eighty percent of what you feed your family is healthy and nutritious, and twenty percent is the occasional cake at a birthday party or dessert after a meal, then you're leading your family toward health and fitness. Not guilt.

Convincing your child to eat right can be a battle. Don't shoot for perfect, shoot for progress—and stay within the boundaries of good health.

Remember the soccer field? We have boundary lines on the soccer field—not so the players can't succeed, but to show the teams that there's a limit or boundary to where you can take the ball. If the ball crosses the lines, everyone stops, and the ball is thrown back within the boundaries again. It's the same thing in eating. Stay in boundary most of the time, but if you eat a brownie or a small bag of chips, enjoy it. Don't eat the whole pan of brownies or two large bags of chips. Enjoy it, and then get back into the game of nutrition so that eighty percent of your family's intake is healthy and nutritious. Use my eighty-twenty rule for eating and you'll always be successful.

Remember: a treat is a treat, and that's OK, but a treat eaten everyday is no longer a treat and can lead to nutritional abuse!

Moms often feel what I call "food guilt" just trying to find the right nutrition for their family in the grocery store. It's hard to say no when your child asks you to buy cookies, ice cream, and potato chips. Let's face it, every food aisle contains treasures and hazards, and you can feel as though you're stepping around landmines to get to the gold. Perhaps no one's told you this before, but we can go crazy trying to be perfect at this! Guilt over food is a self-inflicted stress brought on, for the most part, by the quick-fix dieting concepts. Don't worry over food because someone somewhere said you can't have this or that. Remember—boundaries, not rules! Rules tell you what you can and can't have; boundaries allow you the freedom to eat without guilt!

> **Need to make a quick stop for fast food this week? Check out the best fast-food choices on page 102.**

Eating puts fuel in your body to accomplish your work load for the day. Period. If you like to eat because of the way food tastes, that's OK. If you're hungry, you need to eat, no matter what time of day. But set boundaries for yourself.

What bothers me about the dieting-it-off concept is that we are so focused there, that we don't even know what it is to live anymore. People can get obsessive about food and nutrition until it consumes more time than it should, and it becomes a form of worship. The point of being healthy is to create a balance in your life. Don't make exercise your main theme or nutrition the main theme. Create a balance so they fit into your life so your life is balanced with all the other things—like the work and the relationships that are in your life.

I'd like to tell you one of my television experiences. I was on a television show called *Doctor to Doctor*. The setup of the show is to help the viewer find answers to medical questions by placing five to ten doctors on a panel. We were to answer the questions posed to us. It's live television.

A woman asked the question, "What should I eat if I have diabetes?"

She had ten answers to her one question. When it was my turn, I said, "Let's stop a moment. You're getting ten answers for one question, and your head is probably spinning." I felt as if I wanted to get out of the circle. This woman is pleading in tears, and everyone is pitching their product. Unfortunately, all this information just puts us in bondage. Whom should she listen to? Whom should you listen to?

Here's the short of it. Learn the basics of what you ought to do for health and fitness for your family. If you want to go with South Beach or Dr. Atkins, fine. Take what you know now and follow that information using what I call my eighty-twenty rule. If what you're feeding your family is eighty percent healthy, then you're in good shape. If twentypercent is for taste and fun, that's OK. If you feel twenty percent is too high, then make it eighty-five-fifteen. There is no guilt issue here.

This whole accusation that you're bad if you go off a diet and good if you stay on one is not true. Someone wrote that into eating healthy and ruined it for everyone. Don't go on a diet— problem solved!

If you eat cake every night, you have a problem. But to enjoy one piece of cake is OK. It's OK to have junk food here and there, but don't live on it. Buying food at the grocery store is the same. If the first ingredient is wheat—then probably it's wheat-based. If there's a less desirable ingredient in there, and it's at the bottom, don't worry about it. There's so little in there, it's not going to be detrimental. You want to live healthy and be guilt-free.

> The idea that you're bad if you go off a diet and good if you stay on one is not true.

Think about it. If you want your food to be perfect, you're in the wrong century. The chemicals and pesticides that are in the soils used to grow food today have decreased the value of our food. What are you going to do about that? You can go organic, if you can afford it! You can buy some foods from the farmers' market. But all of it? The spinach we eat today in our salad is not as nutritious as the spinach our great-great grandparents ate one hundred years ago. So, if you really have to be perfect at this and only eat foods that are one hundred percent all the time, then you will need to grow your own trees, plant veggies, and raise sheep so your kids have a perfect lamb dinner when you come home. Do you have time for that?

Probably not. That's why I advise my eighty-twenty rule in nutrition and add a nutritional supplement (multiple vitamin and mineral) to be sure you're getting what's missing in the spinach.

Dump the Junk focuses on educating you by implementing the Fitness Twins:

- Sensible eating habits
- Proper exercise

These will result in healthy, family-friendly lifestyle patterns that you and your family can continue indefinitely.

Dump the Junk!

1. High fructose corn syrup products
2. Fried food
3. Refined flour products

You can lose weight by depriving yourself of food (caloric deprivation) and/or start exercising (increasing your daily energy expenditure). Balancing the two provides healthy life long weight control.

What I have found that works well for most people is to:

- Exercise daily for 30-60 minutes
- Combined with a moderate caloric cutback of 500-750 calories/day.

Before we talk about counting calories, I want to share some simple lifestyle and eating habit changes that can make a big difference in your health and the way you lose pounds.

Ask yourself the following to identify your eating habits:

1. Where are you when you eat?
2. What time do you eat?
3. What is your mood during the meal?
4. How long did it take you to eat the meal?
5. How many activities were you engaged in during the meal? (TV, driving)
6. Who did you eat with?
7. What and how much food was eaten?

> ## Chew food slowly.

Here is a checklist of poor habits and replacement habits in eating. If you see you are checking many of the poor habit boxes, your goal is to eventually replace them with the healthier replacement habits.

Poor Eating Habits	Healthy Replacement Habits
✗ Eat while driving	✓ Eat in the kitchen/ dining room
✗ Eat while watching TV	✓ Eat in the kitchen/ dining room
✗ Don't eat meals at the table	✓ Eat meals at the table
✗ Snack between TV commercials	✓ Drink water between TV commercials
✗ Eat sweets after an argument	✓ Do something physical after an argument
✗ Eat quickly, taking large bites	✓ Eat slowly, take small bites

Poor Eating Habits	Healthy Replacement Habits
✖ Eat foods with extra toppings	✔ Eat foods without toppings
✖ Eat without placing utensils down	✔ Place utensils down after each bite
✖ Eat at different hours every day	✔ Stick to a time schedule
✖ Buy food without reading the labels	✔ Making a set food list before shopping
✖ Eat before going to bed	✔ No eating 3 hours before going to bed
✖ Skip breakfast	✔ Always eat a well-rounded breakfast
✖ Use food to reward weight loss	✔ Buy something new to wear as a reward

Suggestions for proper eating:

- Be a more deliberate eater. Follow a set routine. For example, eat at the same place in the house each day, no matter what you are eating (snack or dinner).

- Use place settings for each meal. Use smaller dishes to prevent overeating.
- Chew food slowly. Chew twenty to thirty times before swallowing. This will speed up the digestive process (enzymatic action). It usually takes fifteen to twenty minutes to satisfy hunger. If you eat a meal in ten minutes, there are still ten minutes left to over eat.
- Set eating utensils down after three bites.
- Initiate conversation between bites.

I hope I have made it clear by now that dieting it off is not an option. America today is the leading nation in the world in diseases and illnesses related to dieting. If you restrict your caloric intake to eight hundred to a thousand calories per day, you deprive yourself of needed nutrients and cause your metabolism to slow down—not what you want if weight loss is your goal.

> **A minimum of 1200 calories is recommended for maintaining good health.**

- Average adult woman: 1,800–2,000 calories
- Average male adult: 2,700 calories.
- Tween and Teenage girls: 2,200 calories
- Tween and Teenage boys: 2,700 calories
- Children: varies based on genetically inherited body type and activity level
- Preschoolers and infants: ask your pediatrician

> **Build a food pyramid sandwich with your kids. See page 87.**

So let's take a look at what often ails us—food. The food pyramid is taught as a part of health curriculum from kindergarten through high school. In fact, you probably remember learning about the food pyramid when you were in school. That's because the food pyramid is a major part of the cement in our childhood foundation for good health. Be sure that you include items from each part of the food pyramid when you shop for food and prepare meals.

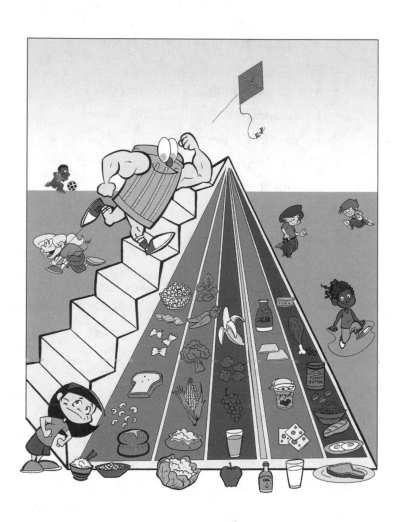

Missing Breakfast

If your child misses breakfast, it will impact his health. He starts off A-OK, but soon starts feeling sleepy and maybe hungry about mid-morning. He is experiencing low blood sugar or hypoglycemia. Both a precursor to diabetes. If there is no healthy lifestyle change, then this child will, because his brain is not nourished, become moody and lethargic and have difficulty concentrating and, worse, experience the onset of diabetes. Due to this condition, his academics and grades suffer. Let's weave this scenario into maintaining a positive attitude throughout life. Ultimately, if this lifestyle remains the same, he will grow up into adulthood without developing the right mental attitude for knowing when he should make changes that would otherwise compromise a healthy life.

> **Plan your meals and
> where you will eat.**

So when should healthy lifestyle changes begin? I say as early in life as possible. It needs to start now with Mom and Dad. Living healthy can become a way of life for them—not a quick fix.

Combating Low Blood Sugar or Hypoglycemia

To lose weight and correct low blood sugar, make certain you include protein in your meals and snacks. Try this simple approach when making your food selections. Combine one protein from below with one or two complex carbohydrates from the Low-Glycemic Index Chart.

Goal: Eat twenty to twenty-five grams of protein per meal or ten to fifteen grams per snack.

Lean Protein (make one selection)

- ☐ 4–6 ounces of chicken or turkey (white meat only)
- ☐ 2 eggs, egg whites or Egg beaters
- ☐ 1 cup of low-fat cottage cheese
- ☐ 4–6 ounces of halibut, sole, cod, scallops, or orange roughy (broiled)

- ☐ 4–6 ounces of lobster or shrimp (boiled) 4–6 ounces of clams (steamed)
- ☐ 4–6 ounces of flounder or haddock (baked)
- ☐ 2 slices of low-fat cheese
- ☐ 4–7 ounces of water-packed tuna
- ☐ 1–2 heaping tablespoons of protein powder
- ☐ 8 ounces of tofu
- ☐ 4–6 ounces of lean red meat (flank or round steak) up to twice per week
- ☐ 1 cup of low-fat plain yogurt
- ☐ 4–6 ounces of salmon (steamed or poached—no sauce) up to twice per week
- ☐ non-fat dairy products with up to 20 grams of protein.

Note: Red meat (lean), oils (canola or olive), nuts and whole eggs are high in fats but in moderation will contribute to fat loss. Eat them sparingly.

Remember it is very important to stay well hydrated preferably by drinking water. Avoid sodas and fruit drinks. Non-caffeine products are best (herb tea rather than coffee). Avoid drinks with NutraSweet or other artificial sweeteners while they don't raise your blood sugar but do stimulate insulin production and can cause hunger.

> If dieting is the silver bullet,
> why is obesity in America at
> epidemic proportions?

Carbohydrates and the Glycemic Index Chart

Good Carbs

These carbohydrates are rated as *low* on the Glycemic Index chart (see page 50) and are called complex carbohydrates. They provide constant energy throughout the day and do not cause you to crash or experience low blood sugar as they do not over stimulate insulin release. Remember them as sort of time-released energy foods.

Complex Carbohydrates

Complex carbohydrates function almost opposite of the carbohydrates rated as *high* on the Glycemic Index chart. They are like time-released energy foods and produce a more constant energy level, which in turn will help stabilize your blood sugar level. This means you can experience constant energy throughout the day without experiencing the *CRASH*. These are categorized as *good* carbohydrates.

These are the preferred sources of energy and should be the main source of foods found in your meals and snacks.

Below is a sample of a Glycemic Index chart. Shown are both types of carbohydrates. Foods are rated by numbers zero to one hundred, with one hundred representing how high the insulin rises when straight glucose (sugar) is ingested. Foods rated higher are high-glycemic or quick-energy foods, such as candy bars, juice, white bread, white rice, corn, and sweeteners such as corn syrup, to name a few.

If you are like most Americans today and get most of your calories from high-glycemic foods, then you are most likely dealing with health and weight problems. To better control your sugar cravings, eat low-glycemic foods as your staples. This will stabilize your blood sugar level and thus promote weight loss. Use the lists for reference when selecting low-glycemic foods.

Do your best to minimize or eliminate high-glycemic foods as they will have the most significant effect on your blood sugar level.

Glycemic Index

Glucose 100

White bread, baked potatoes 95

Honey, mashed potatoes 90

Corn flakes, popcorn, carrots 85

Chocolate bar, candy bar, cookies 70

White rice, refined cereal w/sugar 70

Boiled potatoes, corn 70

Bread (half white, half whole-grain), beets 65

Banana 60

White pasta, jam 55

Brown rice, whole-grain bread 50

Complete cereal (no sugar) 50

Freshly squeezed fruit juice (no sugar) 40

Oat flakes, rye bread 40

Dairy 35

Dry beans, garbanzo beans, lentils, fresh fruit 30

Fruit marmalade (no sugar) 5

Dark chocolate (more than 60% cocoa) 22

Fructose 20

Soy...15

Green veggies, tomatoes, lemon, mushrooms ....<5

High-Glycemic Foods

- Foods containing sugar, honey, molasses, and corn syrup
- Fruits such as bananas, watermelon, pineapple, and raisins
- Vegetables such as potatoes, corn, carrots, beets, turnips, and parsnips
- Breads such as all-white breads, all-white flour products, and corn bread
- Grains including rice, rice products, millet, corn, and corn products
- Pasta, especially thick, large pasta shapes
- Cereals, except those on low-glycemic list below

- Snacks, such as potato chips, corn chips, rice cakes, and pretzels
- Alcoholic beverages

Low-Glycemic Foods

- Foods sweetened with saccharin, aspartame or Fructose and other artificial sweeteners (not preferred).
- All meats
- All dairy (no sugars)
- Fruits, except the high-glycemic fruits listed above
- Vegetables, except the high-glycemic vegetables listed above
- Breads such as whole rye, pumpernickel, and whole-wheat pita
- Grains, including barley, bulgur, and kasha
- Pasta, such as thin strands, whole-wheat pasta, artichoke, and lean threads

- Cereals like Special K, All Bran, Fiber One, and regular oatmeal
- Snacks including nuts, olives, cheese, and pita chips

We know that fat restriction is not the answer to losing and maintaining weight, but rather there needs to be a balance between all the macronutrients—the proteins, carbohydrates and fat.

Let's look at carbohydrates and the Glycemic Index Chart, which is a scale that rates the speed of converting carbohydrates to energy. To keep it simple I'll categorize certain carbohydrates as *bad* and other carbohydrates as *good*, but all carbohydrates are rated on the Glycemic Index Chart.

Bad Carbs

These carbohydrates are rated *high* on the Glycemic Index Chart and are referred to as *simple* sugars. These provide a quick energy boost but are followed by a crash in blood sugar caused by too much insulin release.

> **Eat adequate portion sizes
> from a variety of foods.**

The Blood Type Connection to Diet

We may think that just junk foods are detrimental to our health. But it's actually the common every day foods that may be interfering with your particular biochemistry. Your blood type determines how your body responds to foods you eat. As a proponent of making food selections based on your blood type for accuracy, I want to suggest as you advance in learning the ABCs of healthy eating that you incorporate this approach as a means for personally customizing your dietary regime. (For a complete look at the optimum food selections for your blood type, read my book *Bloodtypes, Bodytypes and YOU,* which can be purchased at www.bodyredesigning.com.)

Here are a few foods that promote weight gain or loss for each blood type:

Blood Type A

- Weight gain: red meat and lima beans
- Weight loss: vegetables and soy products

Blood Type B

- Weight gain: peanuts and wheat
- Weight loss: meats and vegetables

Blood Type AB

- Weight gain: red meat and lima beans
- Weight loss: some red meat, soy products, and vegetables

Blood Type O

- Weight gain: wheat products and cauliflower
- Weight loss: red meat and broccoli

I don't have the space to get too deep into this subject, but the beauty of eating according to your blood type is that losing fat is a natural byproduct. Because you eliminate the incompatible foods from your diet, the toxins once stored in the fat cells will be eliminated. This causes the fat cells to shrink. Need more info? I have it! Please visit my website, www.bodyredesigning.com.

Dietary Supplements

Nutritional supplementation is a must. Contrary to popular belief, even when one tries to get proper nutrition by eating fresh, wholesome, raw foods, they could never receive the same nutrients from these foods that were once possible 40 years ago.

Today's food sources are filled with solvents, pollutants, pesticides, and chemicals in the air. Our once nutrient-rich soils have just about robbed every nutrient.

The diet of the average person today consists of fast-food eating, poor food selections, and poor eating habits. You then can understand the tremendous need for additional nutrients for normal bodily functions and demands.

If that isn't enough, then add one of man's worst enemies today—*STRESS*. Stress is becoming one of the greatest contributing factors to our declining health. These include hypertension (high blood pressure), coronary heart disease, and fatigue.

You must consider dietary supplementation as a safety net for your health. The word *preventative* should be on your lips whenever you defend the importance and value of taking nutritional supplements.

Dietary supplementation is all the difference needed to assist in improving your bodily functions. Dietary supplementation is a preventative measure serving in health protection and as an anti-aging agent that fights against age-related diseases.

Dietary supplementation supports improved wellness, fat metabolism, immune responses, and nutrient absorption and digestion.

A well-rounded daily multiple vitamin and mineral supplement is ideal for kids.

Section 3

Exercise

Power Up!

*Those who think they have no time for bodily exercise will
sooner or later have to find time for illness.*

—Edward Stanley[5]

Section 3

Exercise

Power Up!

HOW OFTEN DO YOU come home from work or the kids come home from school and sit down in front of the TV or computer and not even acknowledge any of your family members? Over an extended period of time this creates distance, isolation, and obesity.

Spending positive time with family members creates a stronger bond, and that's why family fitness is so important.

I think it is fair to say that most people do not like the thought of exercise—at least, that is the feedback I have received from people for many years. This is one reason I have insisted that those teaching my *Dump the Junk Whole-Health Curriculum* for K-4 kids make the exercise and physical activity component fun! (Be sure to check out www.dumpthejunkamerica.com for more information.)

If you dread the thought of exercise, please stick around because there is so much in store for you if you just give it a try. Include exercises in your daily routine. It is not impossible, even if you have a busy schedule.

Exercise as a Routine

1. Write down specific exercise times on your calendar for the week. You're more likely to do it when it is written down.

2. Leave running shoes near your front door. Exercise together as soon as everyone gets home, because once you sit down, you are probably going to stay there, turn on the TV, and eat. Walking with your children at the end of the day is a perfect way to wind down and have some quality time together as a family.

3. Instead of parking close to where you are going, try parking a couple blocks away and walk.

4. Take the stairs instead of the elevator.

5. Use exercise as a stress management device rather than a subject to complain about. Many times the first five minutes of exercise are not the most enjoyable, but as the body warms up, you feel much better and will probably sleep better as well.

6. Get off at the bus stop several stops before yours.

7. If you are close enough, walk, jog, or bike to school.

8. Instead of coffee or soda for your morning buzz, get a natural adrenaline rush by taking a fifteen-minute walk.

Children Watch Their Parents

Your exercise program should have the simplicity and flexibility to be conducted in the privacy of your home or at a health club, whichever you prefer. You don't need complicated or expensive equipment. Most people do not have a lot of time to spare, so keep your exercise program short but effective. Then you will be able to stay motivated for the long haul.

When I was a kid growing up in the suburbs of Buffalo, New York, I remember the path my father drove to work. He was employed at the Bethlehem Steel plant for forty-six years. I remember watching him drive away from the house down to end of street, where he made a left-hand turn. After that, he turned right, passed five stop signs and a signal light, then turned left after crossing four pairs of railroad tracks. After five more miles of straight driving, he turned right into the parking lot of the plant. He walked about five hundred feet to the building, then to the locker room to the same locker where he hung his personal clothes to change into his work clothes, and from there to his work station. He never veered from that routine. Talk about creatures of habit!

I'm sure you can remember routines or habits that one or both of your parents exhibited on a daily or weekly basis. We remember things that engaged our parents' lives and attentions, and our children will look back, remember (and imitate) our efforts to achieve a healthy lifestyle.

> Coronary artery disease is linked to obesity and is becoming more common amongst teenagers.

Our goal? To encourage our children to get up and move! There are many aspects of physical fitness, but this program will focus primarily on three core areas:

1. **Aerobic**—to strengthen the heart and lungs and maintain optimum weight, muscle tone and bone strength.

2. **Weight-bearing**—to increase bone density and strengthen muscle integrity.

3. **Flexibility or Stretching Training**—to promote range of motion in the joints, to cool down after exercise so that your internal machinery has time to recover at an easy pace.

Three Components of an Exercise Program

It is obviously impossible for me to design a *personal* exercise program for you and your child. However, I can give you an idea of what your body requires. All exercise programs should consist of the following three components:

1. Aerobic/Cardiovascular Conditioning

Aerobic/Cardiovascular Conditioning enhances your stamina and endurance by improving your ability to take in oxygen. Cardiovascular conditioning occurs when you remain active at a heart rate of sixty to seventy percent of your maximum heart rate.

Dump the Laziness!

- Unmotivated
- Tired
- Slacker

Exercises

- Walk
- Jog
- Jump rope
- Circuit training
- Stationary bike
- Treadmill
- Elliptical machine

Benefits

- Strengthens the heart
- Strengthens the lungs
- Improves circulation
- Reduces cholesterol level
- Reduces body fat percentage

- Improves ability to recover from physical exertion
- Burns fat

> **More than one in five children ages 6–17 are overweight.**

2. Strength or Resistance Training

Strength or Resistance Training to increase bone density and strengthen muscle integrity. Strength and resistance training will strengthen the muscles and soft tissue that support the joints.

Strength Training Equipment and Exercises

- Multi-station exercise machines
- Conventional machines using cables and pulleys with weight stacks
- Plate-loaded equipment
- Free weights such as barbells or dumbbells

- Isometric exercises
- Negative resistance training
- Gravitational exercises
- Manual resistance exercises

Benefits

- Improves muscle size, shape and strength
- Elevate your good cholesterol (HDL) levels
- Insulin sensitivity improves
- Extended functional independence
- Bones become stronger
- Contributes to lowering the bad cholesterol (LDL)
- Stimulates your metabolic rate for burning fat calories
- Aids in the prevention of injury by promoting proper balance among the various muscle groups
- Improved body composition by increasing the lean muscle tissue and lowering the body fat percent

3. Flexibility or Stretching Training

This type of training enhances and promotes the ability to move a joint through the full range of motion (ROM) without discomfort and relieves stress and anxiety.

Exercises

- Yoga
- Static stretching
- Ballistic stretching—gentle bouncing motion
- Full range of motion for every joint

Benefits

- Relieves stiff joints
- Relaxing
- Promotes elongation of muscles and soft tissue
- Promotes flexibility of muscles and soft tissue
- Decrease in muscle and joint injury and soreness
- Lubricates the dry joint area
- Reduces stress and anxiety

When stretching a muscle, stretch it until it becomes comfortably tight but not painfully uncomfortable. Do not jerk the limbs you are stretching, but simply apply a constant, gentle stretch. Be careful not to stretch beyond that comfort point or you will not be able to relax the muscle and not benefit from the stretching exercise.

I recommend that you warm up the muscles first then stretch them out. For example, the next time you decide to jog or power walk, it would be wise to walk gently for about ten minutes. Warm up those calf muscles by pumping blood into them and lubricate those joints by inducing synovial fluid. Then, after the short warm-up or pre-workout session, take time to stretch the muscles involved in your workout for that session.

Properly stretched muscles will perform at their optimum.

> **It is essential to stay active and exercise a minimum of three times weekly.**

Before you jump into an exercise program, let's look at some basics that need to be addressed regardless of your goals.

Progressive Family-Friendly Fitness Principles

When you read the principles below, remember to stay focused on the purpose and not the task. If you can look back on your week as a family and see that you've made progress, then you've had a winning week! Shoot for progress, not perfection!

Principle # 1: *It's all about the family*. The nice thing about exercising is that it can be social. Get the kids away from the TV, Game Boys, and the Xboxes. Take them outside and play tennis, soccer, or volleyball, take walks, ride bikes, or throw the football around.

Principle # 2: *Exercise for a minimum of fifteen minutes*. Recent research has shown that as few as twelve minutes of exercise per session can produce cardiovascular improvement (stamina but not much fat reduction). To assure more fat reduction, try aerobic training, which is low in intensity and long in duration. Then you will be able to exercise longer.

Principle #3: *Warm up and cool down.* Ideally, a ten-to-fifteen-minute warm-up of walking or cycling prepares the heart, lungs, and muscles for a vigorous workout. It raises your core body temperature, which puts your body into a fat-burning mode. After your workout is over, stretching is a perfect way to cool down.

Principle #4: *Drink water to stay hydrated.* Start out with an eight-to-ten-ounce glass of water about twenty minutes before each workout session. Drink during the workout and immediately after your exercise session. Don't wait until you get thirsty to hydrate.

Principle # 5: *Practice safety during exercise.* Monitor your heart rate (pulse) throughout exercising. Breathe normally. Do not hold your breath—it raises blood pressure. Concentrate on the proper technique and body alignment, especially during weight training.

Wear proper walking shoes for walking, jogging shoes for jogging and tennis shoes for tennis.

Principle #6: *Beware of the heat and humidity.* It is not advisable to exercise in temperatures more than eighty-five degrees with humidity of seventy-five percent or greater. The body has difficulty in cooling itself down, and this could lead to dehydration, heat cramps, heat exhaustion, or even the more severe condition of heat stroke. Clothing should be light and not binding or restrictive.

Principle # 7: *Do a variety of exercises.* Follow a baseline of exercises at least three times per week, but mix it up on the other days. Add recreational activities like biking or hiking. Play some tennis or volleyball. Keep it interesting by varying your activities. Keep moving!

Principle # 8: *Exercise a minimum of three times weekly.* If you exercise fewer than three days per week, you might find it difficult to get fit and lose body fat. On the other hand, you should start out slowly but progressively, allowing only what your fitness condition dictates. Too much too fast will cause potential injury and burnout and will lead to frustration and eventual dropout.

That's SO Random!

Of course, we don't want to get *too* serious! Our children will think we're boring. I want to provide a few "random" exercises (below) that you can do with your child (randomly, of course) that will get them giggling. Be sure to threaten to tickle them if they don't participate in your "random exercise."

Laugh it up! Seriously! According to the Mayo Clinic, laughter releases endorphins, which are said to be a natural pain killer and can actually lower blood pressure, boost the immune system, increase circulation and—well, make you socially compatible with children.

Here's how you play: Declare loudly, "OK, everybody, RANDOM EXERCISE!" Listen to them groan, threaten to tickle them, watch them smile, and then give your child one of these directives:

- **Make the bed.** Hop on one foot (alternating feet is OK).

- **Commercial's on.** Touch your toes twenty times sitting down and then standing up. Last one to finish gets tickled.

- **Folding laundry.** Throw a towel (or a pair of jeans) at them. Hold both ends, one in each hand. Use your own towel to demonstrate. Lift the towel over your head, elbows straight, and stretch left to right, side to side. Go as far as you can without falling or bending your elbows.

- **Coming home.** Before going inside the house together, each family member stands on the outside steps of the doorway, hangs heels over the back edge of the step, and drops heels downward to stretch the calf muscles.

- **Commercial's on again.** Switch off the TV and yell, "Chicken Dance!" Jump up and do the chicken dance (the swim dance, the fishing dance, the soccer dance) with me! Don't know how? Make it up!

- **Putting away groceries.** Hand your teenager two gallons of milk or two containers of laundry detergent (hand your younger child two cans of food). Now have them raise the jugs out from their sides to shoulder level five times and then five times to the front.

- **Pillow fight!** It's the best way to exit all couch potatoes.

So go ahead—laugh it up with your kiddos. And don't forget to tickle.

Physiological Benefits

Exercising your body can be fun. And really, it's not about hard work but rather about being smarter. Whatever your goals for fitness, exercise will be your reliable companion for life. It will never fail you or your child.

> **Focus on the purpose, not the task.**

Let's see what benefits are in store for you:

- **Cardiovascular system**—Heart muscle function is improved by exercise. A conditioned heart is capable of handling physical stress more efficiently and recovers more quickly (improved resting heart rate). A strong heart is more likely to rebound after a heart attack.

- **Circulatory system**—Exercise increases the flow of blood throughout the body, enhances energy, and promotes stamina. It positively affects sexual and mental health and removes toxins from your body. It also nourishes every living cell in your body by delivering with oxygen, vitamins, minerals, and other nutrients.

- **Pulmonary system**—Exercise increases lung capacity, enhances stamina, and endurance. Exercise creates more energy, not less!

- **Digestive system**—This system is improved enormously through exercise, which helps remove dangerous toxicity buildup in the colon. It normalizes bowel movement and greatly enhances regularity and proper bowel function. Exercise also helps with eliminating water retention.

- **Detoxification system**—A natural cleansing occurs as exercise promotes perspiration, which causes your body to rid itself of toxins, water retention, salts, and cellular debris (all toxins).

- **Lymphatic system**—Only exercise detoxifies the lymphatic system and flushes other vital organs.

- **Exercise** helps stabilize the blood sugar level. It allows constant energy flow throughout the day and enhances weight loss.

- **Exercise** promotes healthier skin and skin tone by increasing blood flow closer to the surface skin.

- **Exercise** slows down the aging process by improving mental alertness and prevents or slows down the onset of mental illnesses that are common today, like Alzheimer's and dementia.

- **Exercise** strengthens muscles, ligaments, and cartilage; improves joint mobility and flexibility; and promotes bone density, which prevents the onset of osteoporosis.

- **Exercise** raises your HDL (good cholesterol) and helps reduce your LDL (bad cholesterol). HDL helps remove plaque in the arteries. The net result is a better HDL/LDL cholesterol ratio and a lower risk of heart disease, diabetes, stroke, and a host of other potential medical ailments.

Your threefold metabolic benefit from exercise:

1. Your metabolism is revved during your workout or physical activity, which utilizes stored fat for the energy to perform the exercises.

2. There is an after-burning effect for up to an hour or so after your workout is over, causing your body to continue to burn fat calories after you stop exercising.

3. By developing a positive body composition (increased lean muscle mass and less

body fat) through exercise, your body burns calories more efficiently twenty-four hours per day, which means while you are sleeping, sitting at your desk, or lying on the couch, your body is burning calories—not storing them!

Remember, focus on the purpose, not the task. What more could you want? Sounds like the benefits certainly outweigh the effort to me!

Fun Family Recipes

Yogurt Smoothies

A fruit and yogurt smoothie is a quick and fun way to get more fruit and calcium into your child's diet. Children will need help to make a smoothie, but tweens and teens can be taught to mix a smoothie on their own. Here are some smoothie recipes you may want to try with your kiddos.

Ingredients

- ☐ ½ cup of your child's favorite fruit such as peaches, bananas, pineapples, strawberries, etc.
- ☐ ¾ cup of yogurt
- ☐ 1 cup lowfat milk
  - ☐ Sweetener—avoid artificial sweeteners. Try ¼ cup of frozen apple juice or frozen pineapple juice

Directions

Throw the ingredients into your blender, mix, and serve in a chilled glass with a straw. You may need to add ice or use frozen fruit if you want the smoothie extra cold.

Find a mix that your child likes and try variations of that basic mix.

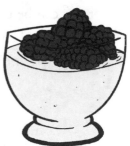

You can find more smoothie recipes at www.smoothieweb.com or simply type "smoothie yogurt recipes" into your search engine and find great ideas there. (See Page 210 of my book *Bloodtypes, Bodytypes and YOU.*)

Healthiest Smoothies

After you find a smoothie mix that your child loves, you may want to slowly introduce variations of healthier smoothies.

- Add protein powder to their smoothies for extra nutritional punch.
- Use nonfat yogurt.
- Keep the skin on when using fruits like apples or pears to get extra fiber.
- Use skim milk.
- Add Stevia (natural sweetener) instead of sugar.
- Add peanut butter for more protein— this works best with a vanilla or banana smoothie.

Yogurt is also a super food, as it contains good bacteria that are important for keeping your child healthy. If your child is lactose intolerant, yogurt might be a good choice. Many people who are lactose intolerant are able to tolerate yogurt, as it is naturally low in lactose, and the bacteria in yogurt help the body produce lactase to digest lactose. If your child has to watch his/her sugar intake, you can try plain yogurt with fruit. Plain yogurt also works really well as a substitute for sour cream in many recipes (e.g., hamburger stroganoff).

Food Pyramid Sandwich

Have you ever built a food pyramid sandwich? That's one of the fun activities included in my Dump the Junk classroom curriculum (available online at www.dumpthejunkamerica.com). Let your child choose one item from every food group on the list below and build a food pyramid sandwich!

Ingredients

- ☐ Whole Grains—Wheat or rye bread, whole-grain bagel, tortilla, English muffin, pita bread, hoagie roll, or bun
- ☐ Vegetables—Romaine lettuce, spinach leaves, cucumber slices, green and yellow pepper rings, alfalfa sprouts, sweet onion slices, mushroom slices, grated carrots, summer squash slices, avocado slices, black or green olives, grated fresh beets
- ☐ Fruits—Banana slices, raisins, applesauce, pine-apple tidbits, blueberries, kiwi fruit slices, straw-berry slices, tomato slices

☐ Dairy—Low-fat ricotta cheese, low-fat cheese (sliced or grated), nonfat plain or fruit-flavored yogurt, low-fat cream cheese

☐ Meat and Beans—Peanut butter, lean sliced turkey, ham, or roast beef, water-packed chunk light tuna, refried beans, thin-sliced toasted almonds

☐ Fats and Sweets—Softened butter, mayonnaise, jam, jelly. (These are not included in the My Fill-Up Food Pyramid but may be added in small amounts.)

Directions

Use ingredients that you have handy or employ your "associate grocery shopper" to help you find those items on your list.

Fruit Kabobs

Make your own fruit kabob. You will need some bamboo skewers and six or seven fresh fruits from the list below. Use a firmer fruit chunk at each end of our skewers to hold the fruit in place.

Ingredients

- ☐ Grapes
- ☐ Strawberries
- ☐ Pineapple chunks
- ☐ Banana slices (thick-cut)
- ☐ Peach or nectarine chunks
- ☐ Watermelon chunks
- ☐ Cantaloupe chunks
- ☐ Kiwi slices (thick cut)
- ☐ Apple dices
- ☐ Papaya chunks
- ☐ Mango chunks

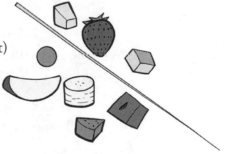

Note to parents: Only provide the amount of fruit that your child will need to prepare one or two kabobs per family member.

Fruits are a good source of vitamin A, vitamin C, and potassium. Vitamin A helps our eyesight. Vitamin C helps keep us healthy. And potassium helps our nerves and muscles to function properly. Did you know there is one fruit that contains all three nutrients? Cantaloupe contains all three. If your child is not a big fan of fruit, see if he or she will eat cantaloupe, and then you will know they are getting all three vitamins. Also, try the fruit-filled recipe below to encourage your child to eat fruit.

Summer Vegetable Salad

Nothing enhances a cool summer salad like bacon and sunflower seeds! You may want to serve the raisins and extra sunflower seeds on the side so that even the pickiest eater will give this dish a try.

Ingredients

- ☐ 5 cups broccoli florets
- ☐ 5 cups cauliflower
- ☐ 2 cups shredded cheese (your choice)
- ☐ ⅔ cup chopped onion (optional)
- ☐ ½ cup raisins
- ☐ 1 cup mayonnaise
- ☐ ¼ cup sugar
- ☐ 2 tablespoons red wine vinegar
- ☐ 6 bacon strips—cooked and crumbled
- ☐ ¼ cup sunflower seeds (optional)

Directions

In a large salad bowl, toss broccoli, cauliflower, cheese, onion, and raisins. In a smaller bowl, combine sugar, vinegar, and mayonnaise. Pour over salad; toss to coat. Refrigerate for 1 hour. Sprinkle with bacon and sunflower seeds. Serve.

Ranch Layered Salad

For the best presentation, layer this salad in a clear glass bowl. Your children can see the ingredients and younger children can count the layers and identify the colors. This salad can also be topped with light mayonnaise and bacon.

Ingredients

- ☐ 1 cup shredded lettuce
- ☐ 1 cup broccoli florets
- ☐ 1 cup cauliflower
- ☐ 1 cup chopped carrots
- ☐ 1 cup fresh or frozen peas
- ☐ ½ cup ranch dressing

Directions

Separate vegetables into individual bowls. Layer each one at a time in a large, clear bowl so layers can be seen. Spoon dressing over the top of the salad. Serve. Yield: 4 servings.

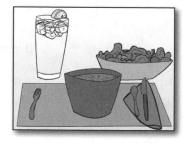

Fresh Vegetable Salad

Is anyone in your family nuts about nuts? Spanish nuts provide protein and enhance the flavor of this summer salad favorite.

Ingredients

- ☐ 6 slices of bacon
- ☐ 3 cups broccoli florets
- ☐ 3 cups cauliflower—chopped
- ☐ 3 cups celery—chopped
- ☐ 1 cup fresh or frozen peas
- ☐ 1 cup dried cranberries
- ☐ 1 cup Spanish peanuts
- ☐ ¼ cup white sugar
- ☐ 1 teaspoon salt
- ☐ 1 tablespoon white wine vinegar
- ☐ 2 tablespoons chopped onion (optional)
- ☐ ¼ cup parmesan cheese
- ☐ 1 cup mayonnaise

Directions

Cook and crumble bacon. Set aside. In a large bowl, combine the next five ingredients. In a smaller bowl, mix together sugar, salt, vinegar, onion, cheese, and mayonnaise. Pour over salad; add nuts and bacon; toss well.

Cool and Creamy Fruit Salad

The texture and taste of lemon (or vanilla) pudding mix combined with small bites of fruit make this a fruit dish that's sure to please your family.

Ingredients

- ☐ 1 20–oz, can pineapple chunks (drained)
- ☐ ½ pound seedless grapes (washed)
- ☐ 2 bananas (sliced)
- ☐ 1 ¾ cups milk
- ☐ 1 small package instant lemon or vanilla pudding mix

Directions

Put the first three ingredients in your bowl and mix gently. Add milk. Slowly stir the mixture while adding the pudding mix. Allow to stand for 30 minutes. Serve.

Banana Sunsicles

Here's a treat you'll want to enjoy outside. Be sure to place this snack on a sturdy paper plate or place several banana sunsicles on a tray over wax paper.

Ingredients

- ☐ ½ banana on a popsicle stick
- ☐ Toasted sunflower seeds
- ☐ Honey (or peanut butter)

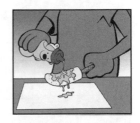

Directions

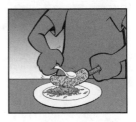

Hold banana by the stick over a piece of wax paper and squeeze enough honey to lightly coat the banana. Roll the banana on the wax paper where the honey dripped to be sure the banana is coated in honey. Pour approximately ¼ cup sunflower seeds onto a clean paper plate. Gently roll the honey-coated banana in sunflower seeds until the entire surface is covered. Use the back of a spoon to pat the seeds onto banana so they really stick. Place the Banana Sunsicle on a clean paper plate.

Pea Pod Surprises

Here's a nutritious treat that your children may want to create. The open pea pod looks like a canoe. How many "people" do you see inside?

Ingredients

- ☐ Chinese pea pods (2 per person, opened along one side)
- ☐ Soft cream cheese

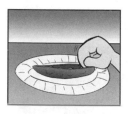

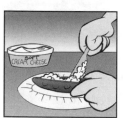

Directions

Using a knife, carefully open one side of the pea pod and spread plenty of cream cheese along the inner surface. Be careful not to open the pod too wide, or it will split, and you will not be able to fill it with the cream cheese. Gently close the pea pod.

Children need to have calcium
to make their bones and teeth
strong and healthy as they grow.
Not all children like to drink
milk, but most will enjoy cottage
cheese and/or yogurt mixed
with other fun foods. The great
thing about cottage cheese is
that it is low in fat but high
in protein. (You can even buy
cottage cheese that is nonfat.)

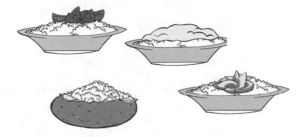

Spinach Dip

Everybody eats chips and dips. They are great party foods. Try this spinach dip with tortilla chips or baked potato chips.

Ingredients

- ⅓ cup real mayonnaise
- 2 ⅓ cups fat-free or light sour cream
- 1 box dry leek soup mix or vegetable soup mix (1.8-ounce)
- 1 cup finely chopped jicama (or substitute a 4-ounce can of water chestnuts, drained and chopped)
- 10-ounce package of frozen, chopped spinach (thaw, drain, and squeeze out excess water)
- 1-pound loaf of sourdough bread (round or similar type)

Directions

In a medium bowl, mix mayonnaise, sour cream, leek soup mix, jicama, and chopped spinach. Chill 6 hours. Remove top and interior of the sourdough bread round, making a bowl. Fill with the spinach mixture. Cut the carved-out bread top into bite-sized cubes for dipping. Yield: About 16 appetizer servings, ⅓ cup of dip each.

Trail Mix

This nutritious blend of fruits, seeds, and nuts can be shared by your family or as a homemade snack for the soccer team. Put the trail mix in snack size zip-lock baggies. Add red and green M&Ms at Christmas and put a bow on your container to create gifts.

Ingredients

- ☐ Raisins
- ☐ Small pieces of dried fruit (pine-apple, papaya, etc.)
- ☐ Raw pumpkin seeds
- ☐ Roasted sunflower seeds
- ☐ Roasted peanuts, soy nuts, cashews, or almonds
- ☐ Mini pretzels
- ☐ Low-sugar banana chips
- ☐ M&Ms (optional treat)

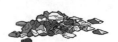

Directions

Scoop ½ cup of each ingredient into the mixing bowl. Mix everything together well before spooning the trail mix into baggies. Store trail mix in the refrigerator. Offer as a quick, healthy snack.

Fill-Up Granola

Granola is great as cereal with milk, a snack by itself, sprinkled on salad, stirred into your favorite yogurt, or even as a topping on frozen yogurt. Here's a new way to enjoy granola in a recipe you'll be sure to enjoy.

Ingredients

- ☐ 10 cups old-fashioned oatmeal (not instant)
- ☐ 2 ½ cups walnuts, almonds, and/or pecans
- ☐ 2 ½ cups toasted wheat germ
- ☐ 1 ¼ cups honey
- ☐ 1 ¼ cups vegetable oil
- ☐ 1 ½ tablespoons vanilla extract
- ☐ 1 ½ cups raisins
- ☐ 1 ¾ cups dried cranberries, papaya, pineapple , or other dried fruit (small pieces)
- ☐ Oil for baking sheets

Directions

Preheat oven to 325°. Lightly oil shallow pans and set aside. In a very large bowl, stir together oatmeal, nuts, and wheat germ. In a medium bowl, mix together the honey, oil, and vanilla. Pour the honey mixture over the oatmeal mixture and stir until blended thoroughly. Spread the mixture onto the baking pans and bake for 15 minutes. Remove pans from the oven and allow the granola to cool. Place granola in a very large bowl. Add raisins and dried fruit and stir until blended. Store granola in an airtight container. Yield: 14 servings

Fast-Food—
Healthier Choices

Subs to Go

Less fit choices	**Healthier choices**
1. White flour bread	1. Whole grain bread
2. 12-inch size	2. 6-inch size
3. Fatty meats such as bacon, ham, meatballs, or tuna salad	3. Lean meat such as chicken, roast beef, or lean ham (or all veggies)
4. High-fat cheese such as cheddar or American	4. Low fat cheese such as mozzarella, Swiss, or provolone
5. Additional mayo or rich sauce	5. Request low fat dressing or mustard
6. Add extra meat or cheese	6. Add extra veggies
7. Kettle cooked potato chips	7. Baked potato chips

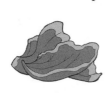
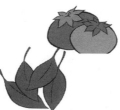
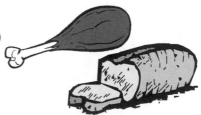

Fast-Food Burger Chains

Less fit choices	Healthier choices
1. Double- or triple-patty hamburger with sauces and bacon	1. Single-patty burger without mayo or cheese
2. Breakfast biscuit sandwich	2. English muffin breakfast sandwich
3. Fried chicken sandwich	3. Grilled chicken sandwich
4. French fries	4. Baked potato
5. Milkshake or sundae	5. Yogurt parfait
6. Chicken nuggets	6. Veggie burger

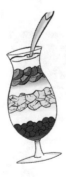 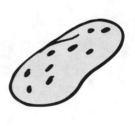

Fried Chicken Food Chains

Less fit choices	Healthier choices

Less fit choices

1. Fried chicken, original or extra-crispy
2. Teriyaki wings or popcorn chicken
3. Caesar salad
4. Chicken and biscuit bowl
5. Adding extra gravy and sauces

Healthier choices

1. Skinless chicken breast without breading
2. Honey BBQ chicken sandwich
3. Garden salad
4. Mashed potatoes
5. Limiting gravy and sauces

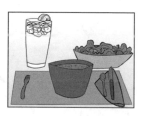

Italian Food Chains

Less fit choices	Healthier choices
1. Pan or thick-crust pizza	1. Thin-crust pizza
2. Extra cheese	2. Extra veggies
3. Buttery garlic bread or oily breadsticks	3. Plain rolls or plain breadsticks
4. Pasta with cheese and meat	4. Pasta with veggies
5. Pasta side or appetizer	5. Veggie side or appetizer
6. Fried entree	6. Grilled or baked entrée

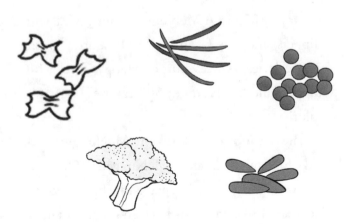

Quick Tips: Fast Food

It should never be your first choice, but sometimes fast food is your only option between driving to soccer practice and ballet. Here are a few tips to help you navigate!

Health magazine rated America's top ten healthiest fast foods. You may be surprised to know that McDonald's made the cut! Sure, Big Macs are still stuffed with calories, but the Golden Arches also serves up a yogurt and granola parfait and a yummy list of salads. McDonald's snack wraps weigh in at 260 to 270 calories each, and their kids' Happy Meals are making moms happy too, with a side of apple dippers instead of fries and low-fat milk or fruit juice instead of soda.

Happy Meals. A McNugget Happy Meal with apple dippers and low-fat milk: 390 calories (with juice, 380 calories). Cheeseburger Happy Meal with apple dippers and low fat milk: 500 calories (with juice, 490 calories).

The Scoop on Chicken McNuggets. McDonald's four-piece Chicken McNuggets: 190 calories and twelve grams of fat. Burger King four-piece Chicken Tenders: 180 calories and eleven grams of fat.

31.9% of children and
adolescents are overweight
and 16.3% of children are
obese in the United States.[6]

Counting Small Fries. McDonald's fries are made with canola-blend oil and have less sodium than Burger King. A small order of fries is just 230 calories and eleven grams of fat. If necessary, split a small order of fries with all of the kids or skip the fries and have apple slices.

Panera Bread. If you have time to run inside, Panera Bread is at the top of America's healthiest fast-food stops. You can choose whole-grain bread and baked potato chips and half-size your order to control portion sizes. Panera serves kids squeezable organic yogurt (70 calories) and kid-friendly deli sandwiches that weigh in at a reasonable 300 to 320 calories each (except for PB&J at 410). Kids gravitate to Panera's grilled organic cheese on whole grain bread.

Fast-food Tips

- Order small—don't supersize (a single patty burger, small fries, and water is about 500 calories; a supersized meal is easily 1,700 calories).
- Order water instead of soda

Best Option: Prepare healthy snacks at home and carry them with you in the car.

Snack Attack

Arm Your Family Before the Snack Attack

Snacks. Everyone needs them. You can arm your family with a warehouse of quick-grab snacks before the snack attack hits. Some snacks such as trail mix or peanut butter crackers will keep well in your van or car, as long as it's not too hot outside. Other snacks can be dropped into a lunch box with an ice pack. Here are some great snack ideas that you can prepare ahead of time.

Snacks to Go

- Sandwich baggies filled with crisp, cut-up vegetables
- A plate of fresh fruit kept in fridge, ready to grab
- Trail mix—usually a base of peanuts and raisins with a variety of dried fruit and nuts (See Page 238 of my book *Bloodtypes, Bodytypes and YOU.)*

- Frozen grapes kept in sealed one-serving containers in the freezer
- Fat-free yogurt or cottage cheese (frozen yogurt in a tube works well)
- String cheese, low fat
- Cut-up apples, strawberries, pears, kept in sealed plastic containers
- Water bottles—It's important to stay hydrated!
- Toasted almonds
- Peanut butter crackers
- Cheese cubes

Three building blocks on which children thrive

Attitude—Think up!

Exercise—Power up!

Nutrition—Fill up!

Remember to shoot for progress, not perfection. And focus on the purpose, not the task. Dump the junk. You can do it!

Epilogue

HAVING SPENT NEARLY MY entire adult life both personally and professionally in helping people of all ages and walks of life be healthy, I let my passion carry over to our youth with a message and instructions for developing healthy lives. Our young people have value and worth in themselves that need to be reenforced, and they need guidance to develop healthy lifestyle standards to live by.

One day your daughter or son may make you a grandparent and even become a future leader in our country. Their beginnings are essential to where destiny takes them, and their physical and mental health is significant to their success.

Now that you have some healthy nuggets in this book to assist you in this cause for helping our kids win the battle against childhood obesity and related illnesses, let me say that this is just our first step.

Dump the Junk America is a part of the solution to childhood obesity and is very passionate about helping our kids be healthier. To be successful, this journey must start at a young age. As a parent and grandparent, I stand with you in this journey to walk the talk and be willing to lead by example!

Endnotes

1. http://www.quotedb.com/quotes/103 (Accessed July 31, 2010)

2. http://www.surgeongeneral.gov/news/testimony/ obesity07162003.htm (Accessed July 31, 2010)

3. http://thinkexist.com/quotation/i_count_him_ braver_who_overcomes_his_desires_than/12815.html (Accessed July 31, 2010)

4. C. Ogden, *High Body Mass Index for Age Among US Children and Adolescents, 2003–2006* (Journal of the American Medical Association, 2008), vol. 299, 2401–2405.

5. http://thinkexist.com/quotation/those_who_think_ they_have_no_time_for_bodily/194816.html (Accessed August 2, 2010)

6. C. Ogden, *High Body Mass Index for Age Among US Children and Adolescents, 2003–2006* (Journal of the American Medical Association, 2008), vol. 299, 2401–2405.

IF YOU'RE A FAN OF THIS BOOK, PLEASE TELL OTHERS...

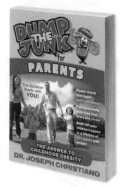

- Write about *Dump the Junk for Parents—The Answer to Childhood Obesity* on your blog, Twitter, MySpace, and Facebook page.

- Suggest *Dump the Junk for Parents— The Answer to Childhood Obesity* to friends.

- When you're in a bookstore, ask them if they carry the book. The book is available through all major distributors, so any bookstore that does not have *Dump the Junk for Parents—The Answer to Childhood Obesity* in stock can easily order it.

- Write a positive review of *Dump the Junk for Parents— The Answer to Childhood Obesity* on www.amazon.com.

- Send my publisher, HigherLife Publishing, suggestions on Web sites, conferences, and events you know of where this book could be offered at media@ahigherlife.com.

- Purchase additional copies to give away as gifts.

CONNECT WITH ME...

To learn more about *Dump the Junk for Parents* and the *Dump the Junk Whole-Health Curriculum* for grades K-4 please visit the below Web sites or call the toll free number.

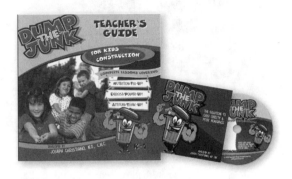

Dump the Junk America offers ancillary educational products and nutrition products for kids. Dr. Joe has created a 501C3 company entitled—*I Care 'Cause I'm Worth It*. It is designed to raise funds for children in furthering their education, careers, etc. To learn more about how you can support our kids, and the Dump the Junk product line, please go to:

www.dumpthejunkamerica.com
or call 1-888-818-6818

For all of Dr. Joe's other books, nutritional supplements and services please go to:

www.bodyredesigning.com
or call 1-800-259-2639

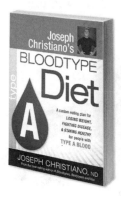
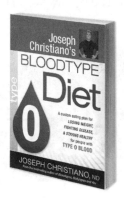